Anti-Inflammatory Diet Cookbook 2023

Recipes for Healing the Immune System, Lowering Inflammation, and Balancing Hormones. Meal Plan for the Next 7 Weeks

Willow Monroe

DISCLAIMER

Every effort has made this book as complete and accurate as possible. This book provides information only up to the publishing date. Therefore, this book should be used as a guide, not the ultimate source.

The purpose of this book is to educate. The author and the publisher do not warrant that the information contained in this book is fully complete and shall not be responsible for any errors or omissions. The author and publisher shall have neither liability nor responsibility to any person or entity concerning any loss or damage caused or alleged to be caused directly or indirectly by this book.

Table Of Content

Get ready

Hello, and welcome to the Anti-Inflammatory Diet Cookbook! The goal of this book is to give you a complete guide to the anti-inflammatory diet, as well as tasty, easy-to-make meals that will help you start on the path to better health without pain.

Inflammation is the body's normal way of protecting and healing itself. But inflammation that lasts for a long time can cause many health problems, like gout, inflammatory diseases, and heart disease. By eating foods that fight inflammation, you can lower it in your body and feel better all around.

No matter how much you know about the anti-inflammatory diet or how new you are to it, this recipe has something for everyone. From energizing breakfast smoothies to healthy grain bowls, tasty dinner meals to desserts that won't make you feel bad, we have a wide range of recipes for you to try.

This book is full of delicious recipes, but it also has helpful information about inflammation, the benefits of an anti-inflammatory diet, and important tips for success. We think that we can take charge of our health and live without pain if we learn about how the food we eat affects us and make decisions based on that knowledge.

We know that beginning a new diet plan can be scary, but don't worry! We've included useful food skills and tips, as well as advice on how to live a life that doesn't cause inflammation. We also talk about common questions, how to fix problems, and how to keep going on the anti-inflammatory diet.

Our goal is to make the switch to a diet that reduces inflammation fun and easy for you. We want you to try out the recipes, change them to suit your tastes, and tell others about your experiences. Remember that this isn't just a recipe; it's a way of life that can change your health and well-being for the better.

So put on your apron, gather your goods, and get ready to go on a delicious and pain-free trip with the Anti-inflammatory Diet Cookbook for Beginners. Your body will be grateful.

Introduction

In the chaos of contemporary life, it is all too simple for our bodies to succumb to inflammation, a silent enemy. Numerous health problems, ranging from joint pain and intestinal discomfort to chronic illnesses like heart disease, diabetes, and even certain malignancies, are caused by this unnoticed foe. But do not worry; you hold the secret to opening a new chapter in your road to bright health and energy inside the pages of this revolutionary cookbook.

Thank you for visiting the "Anti-Inflammatory Diet Cookbook" This literary gem is more than simply a cookbook; it provides a path to a life free from the shackles of inflammation. We are about to go on a gastronomic journey that not only tickles the taste buds, but also calms the body from the inside out.

We'll go deeply into the fundamental nature of inflammation and its complex links to our food in the first few chapters. You'll discover in great detail how certain meals may either feed the fires of inflammation or put out its raging grasp. With this information, you'll learn how an anti-inflammatory diet may be your most effective ally in the pursuit of wellness.

When you start this trip, you'll see it's not about sacrifice or deprivation. It involves opening yourself up to a universe of tastes, textures, and smells that dance pleasantly on your palate and support your body's natural tendency to heal. Imagine indulging in rich but guilt-free treats that tempt your taste buds without sacrificing your health, relishing a substantial bowl of anti-inflammatory soup, drinking a reviving smoothie that is bursting with energy, and so much more.

Each food in this cookbook has been thoughtfully created to incorporate the anti-inflammatory diet's guiding principles without ever sacrificing flavor or enjoyment. We'll look at foods that fight inflammation like gourmet super heroes by being loaded with antioxidants, omega-3 fatty acids, and other nutrients. Each recipe is a celebration of the gifts nature offers to nourish and heal, from the vivid colours of lush greens to the earthy deliciousness of whole grains.

But we don't stop there—our adventure continues. We'll show you how to set up your kitchen, fill your pantry with anti-inflammatory staples, and learn cooking methods that turn even the most basic items into delectable dishes. Meal planning can be made into an art form, and your kitchen may be used as a health testing ground thanks to our professional advice and techniques.

This cookbook is your go-to companion whether you're an experienced food aficionado or just starting out in the realm of mindful eating. No matter where you are in your health journey, you will have the skills you need to succeed thanks to our well crafted meal plans, which are suitable for everyone from beginners to experts.

You'll notice that when you adopt this pain-free anti-inflammatory lifestyle, both your body and mind will benefit. A feeling of thankfulness and awareness that extends beyond the plate will be cultivated as a result of mindful eating activities, which will strengthen your relationship with the food you provide yourself. The advantages spread outward, affecting your general wellbeing and perspective on life.

So come along with us as we embark on this life-changing journey with the "Anti-Inflammatory Diet Cookbook" Turning each page reveals more than simply recipes; it also unlocks the door to a life free from discomfort, overflowing with energy, and paved with delectable intentions for good health. Here is where your path to a pain-free, fulfilling life begins.

Chapter 1:

Foundations Of An Anti-Inflammatory Diet

It is easy to ignore the quiet but powerful force that forms our well-being: inflammation. In a world where the speed of life frequently leaves us feeling permanently harried, it is easy to forget the silent yet powerful force that molds our well-being. The first chapter of our trip through the "Anti-Inflammatory Diet Cookbook" takes us back to the very beginnings of this nutritional approach, showing the route to understanding, battling, and finally overcoming inflammation in order to unleash a life of vibrant health.

What is the Anti-Inflammatory Diet?

Imagine a diet not as a simple collection of foods, but rather as a tactical arsenal that may be used to fight the destructive effects of inflammation. This is exactly what the Anti-Inflammatory Diet is: a way of living that makes use of the power of nutrition to restore harmony to your body, lessen the risk of developing chronic inflammation, and protect you against the adverse effects of a wide range of diseases. It's like a symphony of the best components that nature has to offer, beautifully orchestrated to bring balance to your body.

But what differentiates this eating plan from the other fads and trends that are now prevalent in the health industry? The Anti-Inflammatory Diet, in contrast to transient fads, has its foundation in science and reflects the wisdom of previous generations. It does not place rigorous limitations on you or ask you to make terrible sacrifices; rather, it gives you the ability to make educated choices that feed your body while also calming the fires of inflammation. This dietary philosophy emphasizes the consumption of whole foods that are high in nutrient density and function together in a synergistic manner to provide a holistic approach to wellbeing.

Foods That Trigger Inflammation: A Comprehensive List

We investigate the factors that are responsible for inflammation's smoldering fire. You'll be able to make more educated choices about what you put on your plate after reading our in-depth analysis of a complete list of foods that are known for fanning the fires of inflammation. Sugars that have been refined, trans fats, and eating an excessive amount of red meat are just a few of the common offenders that have been related to inflammation. When you have this information, it gives you the ability to reduce their presence in your diet, which effectively eliminates the factor that is the root cause of many health problems.

Foods That Fight Inflammation: Your Allies in Health

Imagine an army of foods, each one equipped with anti-inflammatories such as antioxidants, vitamins, minerals, and phytochemicals, standing firm against inflammation. We are pleased to provide you with your culinary friends, those foods that have garnered praise for their ability to reduce inflammation. These nutritional powerhouses have the ability to eliminate inflammation at its source. These nutritional powerhouses range from brilliant berries that are brimming with antioxidants to rich fish that are teaming with omega-3 fatty acids. Discover the many benefits and pleasures that come from introducing these foods into your diet, as each bite helps you build a more robust defense against the chronic inflammation that plagues modern life..

Science Behind the Anti-Inflammatory Diet

This dietary revolution is based on science, namely an in-depth study of how our bodies react to the nutrients that we put into our bodies. In this illuminating part, we go into the scientific basis of the Anti-Inflammatory Diet, which will help you better understand how this diet works. Investigate the complex relationship between inflammation and a chain of biochemical events, as well as the surprising capacity of specific foods to halt these reactions, and how the two are connected. Learn how the Anti-Inflammatory Dict may transform your body into a harmonious symphony of health by illuminating the roles that gut health, oxidative stress, and immunological response play in this complex dance of inflammation.

When you commit yourself to learning the fundamental ideas of the Anti-Inflammatory Diet, you are taking the first step on a transforming path that will lead you to a life that is liberated from the weight of pain and enhanced by vitality. The first chapter of this cookbook lays the groundwork for a more in-depth examination of the ways in which ingredients, tastes, and culinary skill might be combined in the following chapters. Therefore, with a willing spirit and a receptive mind, go out into the world and take in the knowledge that will enable you to take command of your health destiny.

Getting Started With The Anti-Inflammatory Diet

We would like to take this opportunity to welcome you to Chapter 2 of your trip through the Anti-Inflammatory Diet in search of a life free from pain and full of vitality. In this part of the book, we will provide you with the foundational skills and information you need to easily incorporate this life-changing lifestyle into your day-to-day routine. We are here to walk you through each step of the process, from transforming your kitchen into a haven of wellness to becoming an expert in fundamental cooking skills.

Section 1: Setting Up Your Kitchen for Success

Your kitchen is not just a place to prepare meals; it's the heart of your journey to wellness. Creating an environment that fosters health and mindfulness is essential for your success with the anti-inflammatory diet. In this section, we'll explore:

Decluttering and Organizing: A clutter-free space promotes a clear mind. We'll guide you through decluttering your kitchen and organizing your cooking tools for maximum efficiency.

Creating a Nurturing Atmosphere: Learn how to infuse your kitchen with positive energy and inspiration. From soothing colors to personalized touches, your kitchen will become a haven for wellness.

Mindful Cooking Space: Transform your kitchen into a space where you can fully immerse yourself in the joy of cooking. Incorporate elements of mindfulness to enhance your culinary experience.

Section 2: Grocery Shopping for an Anti-Inflammatory Pantry

Embarking on an anti-inflammatory journey begins with mindful grocery shopping. In this section, we'll explore the art of curating an anti-inflammatory pantry that empowers you to make nutritious choices effortlessly. Topics covered include:

Essential Anti-Inflammatory Foods: Discover a comprehensive list of anti-inflammatory foods that will be your go-to staples. From colorful vegetables to nutrient-rich grains, you'll learn to select foods that nourish and heal.

Reading Labels: Decode nutritional labels to make informed decisions. Learn to identify hidden additives and sugars that can contribute to inflammation.

Healthy Fats and Oils: Understand the role of fats in your diet and choose the right oils that promote wellness. Dive into the world of heart-healthy fats and their culinary applications.

Section 3: Meal Planning Made Easy

Meal planning is the cornerstone of success in adopting any dietary lifestyle. In this section, we'll empower you to plan your meals strategically and save time while enjoying a diverse and delicious anti-inflammatory menu. Explore:

Strategies for Balanced Meals: Learn the art of combining macronutrients to create well-rounded meals that keep you energized and satisfied throughout the day.

Batch Cooking and Freezing: Discover the magic of batch cooking. We'll guide you through preparing larger quantities of meals and freezing portions for busy days.

Customizable Meal Plans: Delve into sample meal plans that cater to different preferences and dietary needs. Whether you're a vegetarian, a seafood enthusiast, or a meat lover, there's a plan for you.

Section 4: Essential Cooking Techniques and Tools

Cooking is an art, and mastering essential techniques enhances your culinary experience. In this section, we'll cover techniques that preserve the nutritional integrity of ingredients and elevate the flavors of your dishes. Topics include:

Steaming and Sautéing: Explore gentle cooking methods that retain nutrients and flavors in vegetables and proteins. Master the art of sautéing without excessive oil.

Herbs and Spices: Unleash the power of herbs and spices to add depth and complexity to your dishes. Discover their anti-inflammatory properties and how to use them effectively.

Kitchen Tools: From knives to blenders, we'll guide you through the essential tools that streamline your cooking process and enable you to create culinary masterpieces.

Remember that building a solid foundation is key to sustainable change. By setting up your kitchen, stocking your pantry, planning your meals, and mastering cooking techniques, you're not just adopting a diet – you're embracing a lifestyle that nurtures your well-being from within. So, let's embark on this journey of culinary enlightenment and empowerment, where each meal is a step towards vitality and health.

Chapter 3

Breakfasts to Kickstart Your Day

Your morning begins with breakfast, which is more than simply a meal; it's the basis upon which the rest of your day is constructed. In this chapter, we will discuss a variety of delicious morning treats that will not only reawaken your taste senses but will also provide your body with the vitality and nutrition it so desperately needs. These dishes, which range from energizing smoothies to satisfying grain bowls and mouthwatering baked goods, are sure to get you in the mood for an energetic and fruitful day ahead.

Energizing Morning Smoothies

With one of these energizing smoothie concoctions, you'll be able to get your day off to a lively start. These mixtures will stimulate your senses and provide your body with the nutrition it needs to meet the difficulties that lie ahead because they are loaded with antioxidants, vitamins, and fiber.

1. Berry Burst Bliss Smoothie

Serves: 2

Ingredients:

1 cup mixed berries (strawberries, blueberries, raspberries)

1 ripe banana

1/2 cup spinach leaves

1/2 cup almond milk (or preferred milk)

1/4 cup Greek yogurt

1 tablespoon chia seeds

1 teaspoon honey (optional)

Instructions:

Combine all of the ingredients in a blender until they are silky smooth.

Pour into glasses, then top each with a sprinkling of chia seeds for decoration.

Take it slow, relish every bite, and prepare to be flooded with vitality!

2. Green Goddess Power Smoothie

Serves: 2

Ingredients:

1 ripe avocado, peeled and pitted

1 cup kale leaves, stems removed

1/2 cucumber, peeled

1/2 green apple, cored

1/2 lemon, juiced

1 cup coconut water

Ice cubes

Instructions:

Put all of the ingredients in a blender and mix them together.

Blend until smooth, making any necessary adjustments to the consistency with additional coconut water.

Pour into glasses, top with ice, and then savor the deliciousness that is the green liquid.

Bowls of Oatmeal & Grains Loaded with Nutrients

These filling bowls are a celebration of the many different textures, flavors, and nutrients they contain. These bowls are sure to keep you feeling full until your next meal since they are loaded with good grains, protein, and a colorful assortment of toppings.

1. Blueberry Almond Oatmeal Bowl

Serves: 1

Ingredients:

1/2 cup old-fashioned oats

1 cup almond milk (or preferred milk)

1/2 cup blueberries

1 tablespoon almond butter

1 tablespoon chopped almonds

Drizzle of honey

Instructions:

Oats should be cooked in almond milk in accordance with the directions on the box.

Blueberries, almond butter, almonds that have been diced, and a drizzle of honey should go on top.

2. Quinoa Breakfast Bowl

Serves: 1

Ingredients:

1/2 cup cooked quinoa

1/4 cup Greek yogurt

1/2 banana, sliced

1 tablespoon mixed nuts and seeds (e.g., pumpkin seeds, sunflower seeds, chopped walnuts)

1 teaspoon honey

Instructions:

The quinoa, Greek yogurt, and banana slices should be layered in a dish.

Honey should be drizzled on top of the seed and nut mixture before serving.

Wholesome Breakfast Muffins and Bars

These muffins and bars are the ideal grab-and-go snacks for those individuals who are constantly on the move. Because they are not only delicious but also rich in nutrients, they are an excellent choice for a wholesome breakfast even on the most hectic mornings.

1. Banana Nut Breakfast Muffins

Makes: 12 muffins

Ingredients:

2 ripe bananas, mashed

1/4 cup coconut oil, melted

1/4 cup maple syrup

2 eggs

1 teaspoon vanilla extract

1 1/2 cups whole wheat flour

1 teaspoon baking powder

1/2 teaspoon baking soda

1/2 teaspoon cinnamon

1/4 teaspoon salt

1/2 cup chopped nuts (walnuts, almonds, or pecans)

Instructions:

Put a muffin tray in a preheated 350F (175C) oven and fill the cups with paper liners.

Mash the bananas and add them to a bowl along with the coconut oil, maple syrup, eggs, and vanilla.

The dry ingredients (flour, baking powder, soda, cinnamon, and salt) should be mixed together in a separate basin.

Mix the dry ingredients into the wet ones gradually until incorporated.

Mix in the nut pieces.

Scoop the batter into the muffin tins and divide it equally.

A toothpick inserted in the center should come out clean after 18-20 minutes of baking.

Wait till it's cool to eat it.

2. Cranberry Almond Breakfast Bars

Makes: 8 bars

Ingredients:

1 1/2 cups rolled oats

1/2 cup almonds, chopped

1/2 cup dried cranberries

1/4 cup almond butter

1/4 cup honey

1/2 teaspoon vanilla extract

Pinch of salt

Instructions:

Line a baking dish with parchment paper and heat the oven to 350 degrees Fahrenheit (175 degrees Celsius).

Oats, almonds, and dried cranberries should all be mixed together in a big dish.

Almond butter, honey, vanilla essence, and salt are heated over low heat in a small saucepan until smooth.

The almond butter mixture may be poured over the oats and stirred to provide a uniform coating.

Put the mixture into the baking dish and press down firmly.

If you want golden edges, bake for another minute or two.

Bars should be allowed to cool before being cut.

Your mornings will never be the same once you try these delicious dishes. Breakfast is the most important meal of the day since it sets the tone for the rest of your day.

Chapter 4

Nourishing Lunches for Sustained Energy

Lunchtime is a crucial part of your day because it gives you a chance to replenish, refresh, and indulge in energizing, nutritional foods. We'll look at a symphony of tastes and textures in this chapter to make your noon meal more enjoyable. You're in for a treat with everything from zingy salads that are bursting with flavor to warming soups that will warm your heart and creative wraps, sandwiches, and quinoa bowls that redefine midday pleasure.

Section 1: Flavorful, Colorful Salads

Recipe 1: Spicy Chickpea Salad from the Mediterranean

Ingredients:

1 can (15 oz) washed and drained chickpeas

1 cucumber, diced, 1 cup cherry tomatoes, and 1/2 red onion, coarsely chopped

Pitted and sliced Kalamata olives, 1/4 cup

14 cup crumbled feta cheese

14 cup chopped fresh parsley

Olive oil, extra virgin, two teaspoons

Lemon juice, two teaspoons

Oregano, dry, 1 teaspoon

pepper and salt as desired

Instructions:

Chickpeas, tomatoes, cucumber, red onion, olives, and feta cheese should all be combined in a large dish.

The dressing is made by combining olive oil, lemon juice, dried oregano, salt, and pepper in a small dish.

Over the salad, drizzle the dressing and give it a little toss to coat.

Serve with chopped parsley on top.

Asian kale salad with tofu (recipe 2)

Ingredients:

4 cups of chopped and stemmed kale

1 cup of finely sliced purple cabbage

1 julienned carrot, 1 finely sliced red bell pepper

Shelled and boiled 1/2 cup edamame

14 cup of almond slices

8 ounces of diced, sautéed firm tofu

Sesame oil, two teaspoons

Rice vinegar, two teaspoons

a serving of soy sauce

1 teaspoon honey, or, for a vegan version, 1 teaspoon maple syrup

Sesame seeds, 1 teaspoon

Instructions:

Kale, purple cabbage, carrot, red bell pepper, edamame, and sliced almonds should all be combined in a big dish.

Sesame oil, rice vinegar, soy sauce, honey, and sesame seeds are combined to make the dressing in a small bowl.

the salad with chunks of sautéed tofu.

Before serving, drizzle the salad with the dressing, give it a good stir, and then set it aside for a while.

Section 2: Delicious and Filling Soup Recipes

Recipe 3: Butternut Squash Soup, Roasted

Ingredients:

1 medium butternut squash, diced after being skinned and seeded

1 chopped onion, 2 peeled and sliced carrots, and 2 minced garlic cloves

4 cups of veggie broth

1 teaspoon of cumin, ground

1/8 teaspoon cinnamon powder

1/4 teaspoon of nutmeg, ground

pepper and salt as desired

using olive oil to roast

Instructions:

Set the oven's temperature to 400°F (200°C).

Sprinkle salt, pepper, and a splash of olive oil over the cubes of butternut squash. For around 25 to 30 minutes, roast in the preheated oven until fork-tender and slightly browned.

Olive oil and chopped onion and carrots should be sautéed in a big saucepan until tender. Sauté for one more minute after adding the minced garlic.

To the saucepan, add roasted butternut squash, vegetable broth, ground cumin, ground cinnamon, and ground nutmeg. For 15 to 20 minutes, simmer the mixture.

Until the soup is creamy, purée it using an immersion blender. If necessary, season with more salt and pepper.

Serve hot with the option of adding a drizzle of olive oil or a sprinkle of cinnamon as a garnish.

Hearty Lentil and Veggie Soup (Recipe 4)

Ingredients:

1 cup of drained and washed green or brown lentils

two diced carrots and one chopped onion

3 cloves of minced garlic, 2 celery stalks, 1 red bell pepper, and 2 celery stalks

Six cups of vegetable stock

1 teaspoon of cumin, ground

a half-teaspoon of smoked paprika

Bay leaf, one

pepper and salt as desired

For serving, use fresh lemon juice.

Instructions:

To soften the veggies, sauté chopped onion, carrots, celery, red bell pepper, and minced garlic in a big saucepan.

In the saucepan, put the washed lentils, vegetable broth, cumin powder, smoked paprika, bay leaf, salt, and pepper. After bringing to a boil, lower the heat to a simmer, then cover.

Cook the lentils for around 25 to 30 minutes, or until they are soft.

After removing the bay leaf, season the soup to taste with salt and pepper.

Serve hot with a squeeze of fresh lemon juice for a taste boost.

Section 3: Ingenious Sandwiches, Wraps, and Quinoa Bowls

Recipe 5: Hummus Wrap with a Greek Influence

Ingredients:

1 big tortilla made with spinach or whole wheat

1/4 cup finely sliced cucumber and half a cup hummus

1/4 cup finely sliced red bell pepper

1/4 cup finely sliced red onion

1/4 cup of baby spinach or mixed greens

1/4 cup feta cheese crumbles

chopped and pitted kalamata olives (optional)

For garnish, use fresh dill or parsley.

pepper and salt as desired

Instructions:

On a spotless surface, lay the tortilla out flat.

Leaving an inch or so around the edges, cover the tortilla with hummus in an equal layer.

On top of the hummus, arrange the cucumber, red bell pepper, red onion, mixed greens, feta cheese, and olives (if using).

To taste, add salt and pepper to the food.

To make a wrap, fold the edges of the tortilla in, and then tightly roll it up from the bottom.

Add fresh dill or parsley as a garnish and secure with toothpicks if necessary.

Serve after cutting in half diagonally.

Recipe 6: Quinoa and Roasted Vegetable Bowl

Ingredients:

1 cup washed quinoa

2 cups of chopped mixed veggies, including broccoli, bell peppers, and zucchini; 2 teaspoons of olive oil;

1 teaspoon of dried herbs, such as rosemary or thyme

pepper and salt as desired

serving slices of lemon

Instructions:

Quinoa should be prepared as directed on the package and then left aside.

Set the oven's temperature to 425°F (220°C).

Combine olive oil, dried herbs, salt, and pepper with the chopped veggies.

The veggies should be spread out in a single layer on a baking sheet and roasted in the preheated oven for 20 to 25 minutes, or until soft and just beginning to caramelize.

Place a large scoop of cooked quinoa in the center of the bowl to assemble it. Place the quinoa in the middle of the roasted veggies.

Serve with lemon wedges on the side for a tart citrus flavor that will refresh you.

You've started a culinary adventure in this chapter that transforms lunchtime into a celebration of flavor and sustenance. These dishes fill your stomach while also giving your body the nutrition it needs to keep going for the remainder of the day. So feel free to indulge in the flavorful salads, warming soups, and inventive wraps, sandwiches, and quinoa bowls. Your body will be grateful for the food, and every meal will satisfy your taste senses.

Chapter 5

Satisfying Dinners to End Your Day

We examine a variety of filling recipes in this chapter to help you end the day on a healthy note. Dinner is a holy time to nurture your body and spirit. These recipes will transform the way you eat at night, whether it's with lean protein-packed wonders, simple one-pan dishes, or plant-powered treats.

Foods High in Lean Protein

Explore our selection of recipes that are focused on lean proteins to experience the balance of tastes and health. These dishes honor the ideal harmony of nutrient content and flavor, ensuring that your body gets the fundamental constituents it needs for growth and repair.

Lemon-Herb Grilled Salmon (Recipe 5.1)

Ingredients:

Salmon fillets, two

2 teaspoons of olive oil

2 minced garlic cloves, 1 lemon that has been zested and juiced

1 tsp. dried thyme

To taste with salt and pepper

Instructions:

Heat the grill to a moderately hot setting.

Combine olive oil, minced garlic, lemon juice, zest, dried thyme, salt, and pepper in a bowl.

Overspray the salmon fillets with the marinade.

Grill salmon for four to five minutes on each side, or until flaky and thoroughly cooked.

For a full dinner, serve with quinoa or your preferred steamed veggies.

Effortless One-Pan Wonder Recipes

Turn to our one-pan marvels that promise pleasure without the bother on those hectic nights when convenience is paramount. These dishes will change the way you appreciate simplicity in the kitchen since they require little cleaning and have a lot of taste.

Recipe 5.2: Skillet with Mediterranean chickpeas

Ingredients:

chickpeas from one can, washed and drained

a small red onion, finely sliced, and one chopped red bell pepper

Half a cup of cherry tomatoes

1 teaspoon of olive oil

dried oregano, 1 teaspoon

1/8 teaspoon of cumin

To taste with salt and pepper

freshly chopped parsley (for garnish)

Instructions:

Over medium heat, warm up the olive oil in a big skillet.

Red onion and bell pepper, diced, should also be added. to soften, sauté.

Cherries, dried oregano, ground cumin, salt, and pepper should be added. Cook for an additional 2 minutes.

Add chickpeas and stir until cooked all the way through.

Serve as is or over a bed of quinoa, garnished with chopped parsley.

Dinner Favorites Made From Plants

With these plant-powered masterpieces that honor the brilliant hues and flavors of nature, your dining experience will be elevated. These meals will satisfy your hunger and provide you energy since they are full of nutrient-dense components.

Quinoa bowl with roasted vegetables, recipe 5.3

Ingredients:

Uncooked quinoa, one cup

2 cups chopped mixed veggies, including zucchini, bell peppers, and carrots

2 teaspoons of olive oil

one tablespoon of dried rosemary

1/2 tsp. smoked paprika

To taste with salt and pepper

a quarter cup of hummus

Instructions:

Set the oven to 400 °F (200 °C).

Toss the chopped veggies with the olive oil, salt, pepper, dried rosemary, and smoky paprika.

Vegetables should be spread out on a baking sheet, and they should be roasted for 20 to 25 minutes, or until they are soft and have developed a mild caramelization.

Place cooked quinoa in bowls for dishing, add roasted veggies on top, and finish with hummus.

Enjoy the plant-powered deliciousness and if wanted, sprinkle with more herbs or seeds.

Your day should come to a gratifying conclusion with a meal that promotes your wellbeing and boosts your spirits. Whether you choose the protein-packed greatness, the ease of one-pan miracles, or the vivid embrace of plant-powered treats, these dishes are your entryway to changing your evening meals into really nutritious experiences. Good food!

Chapter 6:

Wholesome Snacks for On-the-Go

As we look at many possibilities to keep you fueled and energetic throughout your hectic days, snacking takes on a new level of sophistication. Say goodbye to mindless snacking and welcome these nutrient-rich concoctions that are both tasty and practical.

Nut and Seed Blends for Boosted Energy

These nut and seed mixtures are your on-the-go source of lasting energy, whether you're tackling a hiking path or pushing through a workday. They are the ideal blend of flavor and vitality since they are loaded with beneficial nutrients, healthy fats, and a delightful crunch.

Ingredients:

one cup of raw almonds

walnuts, 1 cup

one cup of pumpkin seeds

a cup of cashews

a half-cup of raisins or cranberries that have been dried

a tsp. of sea salt

half a teaspoon of cumin powder

Paprika, 1/2 tsp.

(Adjust to taste) 1/4 teaspoon cayenne pepper

Instructions:

Set the oven to 325 °F (165 °C).

All the nuts and seeds should be combined in a big dish.

Combine the cayenne pepper, paprika, cumin, and sea salt in a separate small bowl.

Olive oil should be added, and the nut and seed mixture should be well coated.

After thoroughly swirling to achieve uniform distribution, sprinkle the spice mixture over the nuts and seeds.

On a parchment paper-lined baking sheet, spread the ingredients out.

When the nuts are toasty and aromatic, roast in the preheated oven for 15-20 minutes, stirring once or twice.

Before adding raisins or dried cranberries, take the dish out of the oven and allow it cool fully.

For a maximum of two weeks, keep in an airtight container.

Veggie and Dip Combos without the Guilt

The best guilt-free eating is dipping crunchy veggies in delicious sauces. These combinations are not only delicious but also packed with vitamins, minerals, and antioxidants that promote your general health.

Combo 1: Hummus with baby carrots

Combo 2: Paprika sprinkled on top and drizzled with olive oil

Greek yogurt dip with dill and sliced cucumbers

Combo 3: Guacamole with lime juice and bell pepper strips

Combo 4: Snap peas with a lemon-tahini dip Recipe:

Slice or chop the veggies into snack-size pieces after washing and preparing them.

On a plate or in a snack container, arrange the veggies.

Prepare thc dip(s) by either preparing them from home using your preferred recipes or by purchasing prepared choices from the supermarket.

To enhance the tastes, drizzle some olive oil, add some herbs or spices, or juice some citrus.

Enjoy your guilt-free snack assault while eating the vegetables with the dips on the side.

Making Energy Bars and Bites at Home

There is no need for store-bought energy bars that include additives. Make your own healthy versions with plenty of all-natural ingredients to give you a boost of energy anytime you need it.

Ingredients:

Rolling oats in a cup

Almond, peanut, or your preferred nut butter, 1/2 cup

A quarter cup of maple syrup or honey

Nuts like almonds, walnuts, or pistachios, in the amount of 1/2 cup, chopped

if big, 1/4 cup chopped dry fruit (dates, raisins, or apricots)

Cacao nibs or dark chocolate chips, 1/4 cup (optional)

one teaspoon of vanilla extract

Add a dash of salt

Instructions:

Combine the rolled oats, chopped nuts, dried fruit, and chocolate chips (if using) in a large bowl.

Mix the nut butter, honey, and maple syrup well in a small saucepan over low heat.

Take the mixture off the heat, then add a dash of salt and vanilla essence.

When everything is well combined and covered, pour the nut butter mixture over the dry ingredients.

Put parchment paper in the bottom of a baking dish, then pack the mixture down firmly.

Put the mixture in the fridge for at least a couple of hours to let it solidify.

Cut the finished product into bars or bite-sized pieces.

Refrigerate for up to two weeks in an airtight container.

With these filling and nutritional snack suggestions, you have the means to fend off hunger without straying from your anti-inflammatory lifestyle commitment and live pain-free. Enjoy these alternatives for on-the-go eating without giving anything up, and savor the vigor they provide to your day.

Chapter 7:

Flavorsome Sauces, Dressings, and Condiments

Your kitchen's hidden heroes are the condiments, dressings, and sauces you use. They have the extraordinary ability to elevate your meals to new levels by turning a straightforward dish into a masterpiece of tastes and textures. We'll go into the technique of creating these crucial components in this chapter, giving your anti-inflammatory dining experience a special touch.

Section 1: Homemade Sauces to Make Your Meals Better

Discover how to make enticing sauces that bring out the best in each meal. Each mouthful of your meals will be an amazing experience because to the layers of complexity and depth added by these handcrafted creations.

Recipe 1: Romesco Sauce with Roasted Red Peppers.

Ingredients:

2 roasted and peeled red bell peppers

12 cup toasted almonds

2 minced garlic cloves

Extra virgin olive oil, 1/4 cup

Red wine vinegar, 2 teaspoons

smoked paprika, 1 teaspoon

pepper and salt as desired

Instructions:

Roasted red peppers, toasted almonds, minced garlic, smoked paprika, red wine vinegar, salt, and pepper should all be put in a food processor.

The mixture should be well blended yet somewhat lumpy after a few pulses.

As the machine is working, add the extra virgin olive oil in a slow, steady stream until the sauce is the right consistency.

If necessary, taste and adjust the seasoning.

Place the Romesco sauce in a container and cool. It can be kept for up to a week in storage.

Recipe 2: Avocado Basil Cream Sauce

Ingredients:

Peeled and pitted avocado, 1

1 cup of basil leaves, fresh

14 cup roasted pine nuts

Lemon juice, two teaspoons

14 cup of water

Olive oil, extra virgin, two teaspoons

To taste, add salt and pepper.

Instructions:

Avocado, basil leaves, toasted pine nuts, lemon juice, water, salt, and pepper should all be combined in a blender or food processor.

If extra water is required to obtain the desired consistency, blend until the mixture is smooth and creamy.

Drizzle the extra virgin olive oil in while the mixer is running.

When required, taste and adjust the seasoning.

Put the avocado basil sauce in a jar and store it in the fridge. To get the finest taste and freshness, eat within 3–4 days.

Section 2: Multipurpose Dressings for All Salads

Dressings that are bursting with flavor and provide the ideal harmony of acidity and richness may elevate your salads. These dressings, which range from creamy emulsions to zingy vinaigrettes, will elevate your greens to a new level.

Recipe 3 Balsamic Dijon Vinaigrette.

Ingredients:

Balsamic vinegar, 1/4 cup

Dijon mustard, two teaspoons

1 minced garlic clove.

Extra virgin olive oil, half a cup

One teaspoon of optional honey

To taste, add salt and pepper.

Instructions:

Balsamic vinegar, Dijon mustard, minced garlic, and honey (if used) should be combined in a bowl.

Extra virgin olive oil should be added gradually while rapidly whisking to create an emulsion.

To taste, add salt and pepper to the food.

Vinaigrette may be kept in the refrigerator for up to two weeks after being transferred to a glass jar.

Recipe 4: Creamy Tahini Lemon Dressing

Ingredients:

Tahini, 14 cup

Lemon juice, two teaspoons

2 tablespoons of water and 1 chopped garlic clove

1/8 teaspoon cumin powder

pepper and salt as desired

Instructions:

Mix the tahini, water, lemon juice, minced garlic, and ground cumin in a small bowl.

Add extra water if the dressing is too thick until you have the required consistency.

To taste, add salt and pepper to the food.

Drizzle it over your favorite salads or keep it in the fridge for up to a week in an airtight jar.

Flavor-Boosting Condiments You'll Love in Section 3

With these flavor-enhancing condiments, you can transform regular meals into amazing concoctions that give your food a blast of flavor and excitement. These condiments are your hidden weapons for culinary genius, from spicy salsas to fragrant pestos.

Fresh Mango Salsa (5th recipe)

Ingredients:

Peeled and sliced one ripe mango.

12 a red onion, cut coarsely.

1 jalapeño, coarsely chopped with the seeds removed.

14 cup chopped fresh cilantro.

1 lime's juice

Salt as desired

Instructions:

Diced mango, red onion, jalapeño, and cilantro should all be combined in a bowl.

Pour lime juice over the ingredients and toss just enough to incorporate.

To taste, add salt to the dish.

Before serving, let the flavors 15 minutes to mingle. Serve as a dip with whole-grain chips, grilled meats, salads, or other foods.

Basil Walnut Pesto Recipe 6

Ingredients:

2 cups of basil leaves, fresh

12 cup toasted walnuts

1/2 cup grated Parmesan cheese (or vegan nutritional yeast)

Garlic cloves, two

Extra virgin olive oil, half a cup

lemon juice from one

To taste, add salt and pepper.

Instructions:

Fresh basil leaves, roasted walnuts, grated Parmesan cheese (or nutritional yeast), and garlic are all combined in a food processor.

To finely chop the items, continue to pulse.

Extra virgin olive oil should be added gradually while the processor is running until the pesto has the required consistency.

Pulse a couple more times to blend after adding the salt, pepper, and lemon juice.

Put the basil-walnut pesto in a glass jar and put it in the fridge. For best taste, use within a week after purchase.

These condiments, dressings, and sauces are the key to a vast array of culinary options. You'll discover that even the most straightforward foods can be turned into gourmet concoctions that titillate your taste buds and nourish your body as you experiment with various combinations and tastes. Learn to make sauces, dressings, and condiments, and you'll see how your food takes on tastes you never imagined it could.

Chapter Eight:

Sweet Treats without the Guilt

We'll look into the realm of sweet delight that doesn't jeopardize your dedication to an anti-inflammatory lifestyle. These dishes, which range from fruity treats to indulgent chocolate desserts, will sate your appetites while reducing inflammation. Prepare to indulge in a range of guilt-free treats that will make your taste senses dance and your body grateful.

Yummy Fruit-Based Desserts

1. A parfait of berries

Ingredients:

(Strawberries, blueberries, and raspberries)

(Dairy or vegan) Greek yogurt

maple syrup or unprocessed honey

Granola (choose a low-sugar kind)

Instructions:

Stack mixed berries in the bottom of a glass.

Greek yogurt should be spooned on top of the fruit.

Add a little raw honey or maple syrup.

For crunch, sprinkle over some granola.

Layers are repeated, and the final touch is a berry. Enjoy!

2. A salad of tropical fruits and mint

Ingredients:

Sliced fresh mint leaves, lime juice, pineapple, cubed mango, cubed papaya, cubed kiwi, and cubed papaya

Instructions:

In a dish, mix all the fruit pieces.

To enhance the tastes of the fruit, squeeze lime juice over it.

Add chopped mint leaves and stir gently.

Before serving, let the food cool in the fridge.

Anti-inflammatory alterations to baked goods

3. Blueberry Muffins with Almond Flour

Ingredients:

Coconut flour

arrowroot powder

eggs salt

Coconut lard

pure honey

vibrant blueberries

Instructions:

Then, line a muffin pan with liners and preheat the oven.

Combine almond flour, baking soda, and a dash of salt in a basin.

Whisk the eggs, raw honey, and coconut oil in a another bowl.

After combining the dry and wet ingredients, carefully fold in the blueberries.

Bake the dough in muffin tins after dividing it evenly till browned.

4. Bread with Spiced Carrot and Zucchini

Ingredients:

grated zucchini with carrots

(Or flour that is gluten-free) Whole wheat

soda bread

(Ground) cinnamon, nutmeg, and ginger

a vegan alternative would be flax eggs.

the oil of olives

coconut nectar

Instructions:

Set the oven to pre-heat, then butter a loaf pan.

Combine dry ingredients with shredded carrots and zucchini.

Eggs, coconut sugar, and olive oil should be whisked in a separate bowl.

Mix the dry and wet ingredients together, then pour into the pan.

Bake until a toothpick is removed clean.

Chocolate Creations that are Indulgent but Healthy

5. Avocado Mousse with Dark Chocolate

Ingredients:

Fruitful avocados

Inky cocoa powder

Honey or maple syrup

Vanilla essence

Salt shaker-full

Topping with fresh berries

Instructions:

Blend avocados with the sugar, vanilla, salt, and cocoa powder.

The mixture should be refrigerated for an hour.

Add fresh berries on top after ladling into serving glasses.

6. Nut-crusted strawberries in chocolate

Ingredients:

dried and cleaned fresh strawberries

70% cocoa or more dark chocolate

Almonds, pistachios, and other nuts, chopped

Instructions:

Melt dark chocolate in a double boiler or microwave.

Melted chocolate should be used to partially dunk strawberries.

The dipping piece is rolled in chopped nuts.

Place on a tray with parchment paper to cool.

Enjoy these treats guilt-free while letting your taste buds experience the harmonious blending of tastes and advantages to your health. These dishes serve as both a tribute to the anti-inflammatory diet's creative potential and a celebration of the pleasure that comes from feeding both your body and spirit.

Chapter Nine

A Week of Anti-Inflammatory Meal Plans

To help you navigate a week of delicious anti-inflammatory food, we provide carefully developed meal plans. These meal plans are designed to accommodate a range of tastes and degrees of dedication. No matter whether you're a beginner looking for a jumpstart into the realm of anti-inflammatory bliss, someone searching for a gradual shift, or a creative spirit anxious to build your meal plan, we have you covered.

Meal Plan for Novice Foodies for 7 Days

Day 1:

Breakfast: an energizing spinach and berry smoothie

Quinoa salad for lunch, along with roasted vegetables and chickpeas

Hummus with sliced cucumber for a snack

Dinner will be baked salmon, broccoli, and quinoa.

Day 2:

Breakfast: Chia Seed Pudding with Mixed Berries from the previous night.

Lunch will consist of a spinach and kale salad with grilled chicken, avocado, and a lemon-tahini dressing. For a snack, there will be mixed nuts and dried fruits.

Dinner will be a lentil and vegetable stew served with brown rice.

Day 3:

Breakfast would consist of an almond granola parfait with fresh fruit.

Lunch: Whole Grain Tortilla Wrapped with Roasted Vegetables

Snack: Guacamole-topped carrot sticks.

Dinner will be grilled turkey burgers with fries and mixed greens.

Day 4:

Breakfast: Scrambled eggs with tomatoes and spinach

Lunch consists of grilled shrimp and apple slaw.

Almond butter-topped rice cakes as a snack.

Dinner will be tofu in a stir-fry with broccoli and quinoa.

Day 5:

Breakfast consists of sliced bananas, chopped nuts, and oatmeal.

Mediterranean chickpea salad with feta cheese for lunch

Snack: Peanut butter-topped apple slices.

Dinner will be baked chicken with cauliflower rice and roasted Brussels sprouts.

Day 6:

Smoothie bowl with mixed greens and tropical fruits for breakfast

Lunch will be a bowl of brown rice with black beans, salsa, and avocado.

Trail Mix with Seeds and Dried Cranberries as a Snack

Quinoa with grilled vegetable and portobello mushroom skewers for dinner

Day 7:

Breakfast: Poached eggs and mashed avocado over whole-grain toast.

Vegetable and Tofu Stir-Fry with a Thai Influence for Lunch

Bell pepper strips with hummus as a snack

Dinner will be baked fish with asparagus and mashed cauliflower.

Meal Schedule for a 14-Day Transition

This 14-day plan offers a well-balanced introduction to a world of healthy options for people who are just starting out with an anti-inflammatory diet. If you have a preference, feel free to change the components and portion sizes.

Week 1:

Follow the beginner foodies' seven-day meal plan.

Week 2:

Increase the number of plant-based meals you eat, such as grain bowls, stir-fries with tofu, and lentil soups.

To enhance flavor without using salt, experiment with various herbs and spices.

Customizable Meal Planning Strategies

For the creative and adventurous souls, this section empowers you to craft your anti-inflammatory meal plans based on your taste, dietary needs, and schedule.

Choose Your Protein: Mix and match lean proteins like fish, poultry, tofu, legumes, and nuts.

Vibrant Vegetables: Opt for a rainbow of veggies to maximize nutrient intake.

Smart Carbs: Embrace whole grains, sweet potatoes, and legumes for sustained energy.

Healthy Fats: Include sources like avocados, olive oil, and nuts for their anti-inflammatory properties.

Snack Sensibly: Keep nutrient-dense snacks on hand for moments of hunger.

Hydration and Herbal Teas: Stay hydrated with water, herbal teas, and infusions.

Mindful Eating: Prioritize mindful eating, savoring every bite and honoring your body's signals.

Keep in mind that these menus are just suggestions. Making your own delectable and wholesome meals will become more enjoyable as you get more acquainted with the anti-inflammatory diet's guiding principles. Your plate is your canvas as you embark on the path to vibrant wellbeing, which is as individual as you are. Enjoy the process of feeding your body and take full advantage of your anti-inflammatory journey.

Chapter 10:

Maintaining Your Anti-Inflammatory Lifestyle

Maintaining the newly discovered equilibrium and vigor that the anti-inflammatory diet has bestowed upon you might seem like a herculean task in the complex maze that is our contemporary world, where stress and temptations appear to wait around every bend. But don't be afraid because this chapter will act as your compass, guiding you through the twists and turns of life while also providing you with the tools you need to protect the life-altering changes you've chosen to accept. We've arrived to the end of our trip, and with it comes the culmination of our wisdom: "Maintaining Your Anti-Inflammatory Lifestyle."

Conquering Obstacles and Maintaining Your Motivation Throughout Your Journey Beyond Adversity

We are all well aware of the fact that life is full with obstacles. There are times when the pressures of work, family life, and unanticipated events might pose a risk to the foundations of our good behaviors. But keep in mind that the key to enduring transformation is your ability to remain resilient. On the following pages, you will discover a veritable treasure trove of tactics and insights that will allow you to sail even the most turbulent waters.

Acquire the ability to detect the telltale symptoms of diversions that may take you away from the road that will reduce inflammation in your body. Learn the fine art of preparation, whether that means keeping wholesome food on hand for when you're faced with a hectic day or creating a support network that boosts you up. This section is your toolbox for tenacity; it includes everything from the anecdotes of people who have overcome challenges to the research that explains how habits are formed.

The impact that mindful eating has on inflammation: savoring every bite and finding healing from the inside out

Consuming food in a mindful manner is more than simply a passing fad; it's an art form that may have a significant influence on one's overall health. In this section, we investigate the intricate relationship that exists between your senses and the food that you take into your body. You will acquire the skill of savoring each mouthful, not just for the tastes it entails, but also for the nutrients it provides for your body as a whole.

By practicing mindful eating, you'll develop a relationship with the food you consume that goes beyond its function as a source of nutrition. Find out how slowing down and engaging your senses may truly have an effect on how well your body digests food and absorbs nutrients. When you grasp the significant impact that your ideas and feelings have on the formation of your health, science and intuition come together. Prepare to discover the transforming potential that lies inside each lunch ritual.

Wellness from the Ground Up: Sowing the Seeds for Long-Term Benefits and Enduring Health

In this last part of the book, we take a look into the horizon of your future, a future in which vitality is not only a passing moment but rather a continuous companion. The anti-inflammatory diet is not a fad; rather, it is an investment that should be made for the rest of your life in your health and happiness. Investigate the scientific web that links together the advantages that will accrue to you over the course of your trip to reduce inflammation.

Explore the intriguing realm of anti-aging medicine and the art of living a long and healthy life. The decisions you make today will resonate across the years, having an effect on everything from the health of your heart to the quality of your cognitive functioning. Learn how the anti-inflammatory diet may help nourish your cells, boost your immune system, and ultimately promote your overall health and wellbeing.

As we come to the end of this life-changing journey, it is important to keep in mind that you are the creator of the story that is still being written about your life. The knowledge, skills, and recipes that may be gained through reading this book are only the beginning of the journey. You are on the verge of living a life that is abundant with health and satisfaction because you are armed with information, strengthened by experience, and fueled by the desire for vitality.

You are holding more than a cookbook; rather, you are holding a roadmap to living a life that shines with vitality. Now is the moment to embrace your trip with unyielding purpose, to relish each mouthful with intention, and to march on into the future with the bright spirit that you have developed. The journey toward preserving your anti-inflammatory way of life is a holy one, and it is up to you to travel it with a sense of purpose and happiness.

Conclusion

As we approach the conclusion of the "Pain-Free Anti-Inflammatory Diet Cookbook for Beginners," I am overcome with thankfulness and optimism. This trip that we've taken together is more than just a collection of cooking tips and recipes; it's a monument to your dedication to taking care of yourself and your unwavering determination to live a healthy life.

You've learned more about anti-inflammatory nutrition than simply the foods to consume and stay away from as a result of your research. You now have the ability to make decisions that will affect every aspect of your health. You have developed a knowledge of the complex relationship between food and inflammation, as well as how the meals you choose may either promote vitality or cause pain.

Keep in mind that this is an ongoing transformative effort that will have lasting effects. The knowledge you've gained in these pages is intended to be used outside of the kitchen. They will help you navigate the grocery store aisles, influence your restaurant menu decisions, and serve as inspiration for your future food preparations.

An anti-inflammatory dinner is being enjoyed as you indulge in self-love. Your body is getting the nutrition it needs, and your spirit is getting tastes that make you happy. This is a celebration of life's plenty and your persistent dedication to using it for your well-being rather than only food.

I want you to continue the author-reader collaboration that has existed throughout your experience with this cookbook. As you explore new ingredients, try out new flavors, and modify recipes to fit your own tastes, let curiosity be your guide. Enjoy being creative in the kitchen knowing that your decisions are in line with your health objectives.

There will always be obstacles, and there will be moments when convenience appears to trump purpose. Recall the benefits of mindful eating and the experience of your journey at these times. Keep in mind that every decision you make is a chance to invest in your health, and that this investment will pay you in the form of continued vitality and a life free from pain.

Knowing that your trip is far from done as you digest the last bits of knowledge from this book. The path ahead is one of ongoing development, discovery, and change. Discover new tastes, seek out new recipes, and give the gift of your newly acquired knowledge to loved ones. By doing this, you greatly increase the impact of health and happiness outside of your own life.

I am privileged to have served as your guide on your journey to a pain-free, fulfilling life. Together, we have been on a path of self-discovery, personal growth, and health passion. As you put this book away, keep in mind that the decisions you make today will determine how vibrant and joyful your future will be. The choices are as boundless as the tastes waiting to be experienced as your trip has only just started.

with sincere gratitude and unwavering faith in your ability.

9 798867 447564